Crohn's Disease

All You Need to Know

Disclaimer

This content serves to provide general information about the disease and aims to empower you to seek prompt medical assistance if necessary to prevent complications. It's essential to stress that this information is not a substitute for consulting a qualified physician. The field of medical science is continually evolving, and due to the dynamic nature of medical knowledge, we recommend seeking expert advice if you encounter any inconsistencies or intend to take action based on the information in this content. Never disregard professional medical guidance or delay treatment based on something you've read online, including this material, or from any other online source. Always remember that the internet cannot cure you; rather, healing comes through the guidance of medical professionals and the providence of God.

Table of Content

Introduction

Information on possible causes, symptoms, treatment options, and general management of Crohn's disease is provided in this article.

A persistent inflammatory disorder of the gastrointestinal system is called Crohn's disease. You and your loved ones can better manage the uncertainty that accompanies a new diagnosis if you and they understand Crohn's disease.

Crohn's disease is a member of the inflammatory bowel disease, or IBD, category of illnesses. It bears the name of Dr. Burrill B. Crohn, who, along with Drs. Leon Ginzburg and Gordon D. Oppenheimer, initially described the disease in 1932.

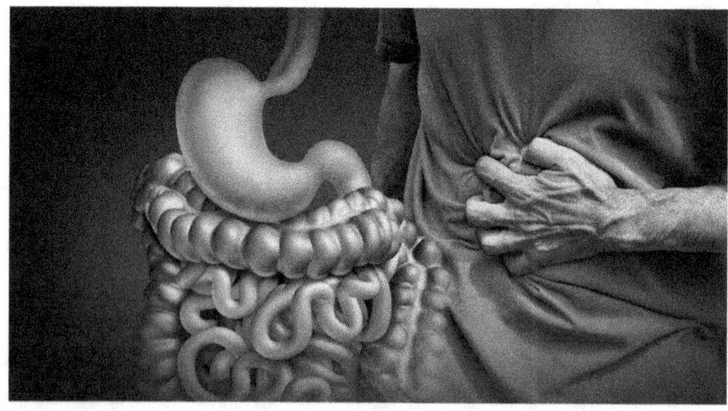

Key Fact

- There is an equal chance for men and women to be impacted.
- Although Crohn's disease can strike anyone at any age, it is most common in adults and adolescents between the ages of 15 and 35.
- Stress and diet can exacerbate Crohn's disease, but they do not cause it.
- According to recent studies, environmental, genetic, and familial variables all play a role in the development of Crohn's disease.

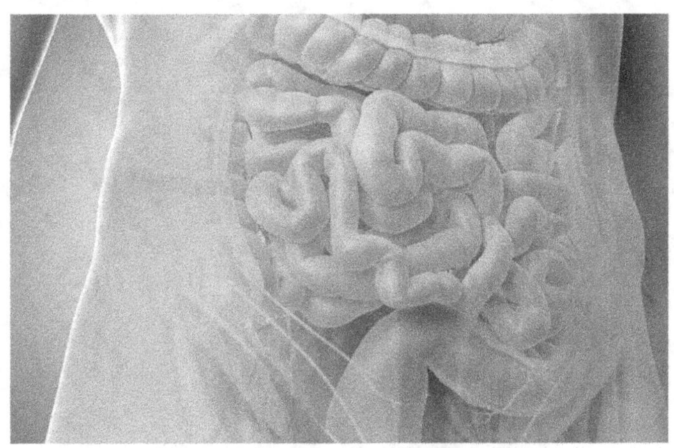

**Gastrointestinal system
Having Swollen Colon - Large Intestine**

Crohn's Disease vs. Ulcerative Colitis

Although Crohn's disease and ulcerative colitis are both forms of inflammatory bowel disease (IBD) and have similar symptoms, they are distinct illnesses that affect separate parts of the GI tract.

Crohn's disease
- can impact the mouth, anus, and any portion of the GI system.
- can impact the gut wall's total thickness.

Ulcerative colitis
- The colon and rectum—also referred to as the big intestine—are the only organs impacted.
- impacts the big intestine's interior lining.

Section 1

Who Can Be Affected?

- It is estimated that 1 in 100 Americans have IBD. Crohn's disease is equally likely to affect males and women.
- Although Crohn's disease can strike anyone at any age, it is most frequently identified in adults and teenagers between the ages of 20 and 30.
- According to studies, between 1.5% and 28% of persons with IBD have a first-degree relative—a parent, child, or sibling—who also has the illness.
- Despite a hereditary component linked to an elevated risk of IBD, family history cannot be used to predict who would get Crohn's disease.
- People with Crohn's disease might be of any ethnicity. Although prevalence of Crohn's disease among Asians and Hispanics have increased recently, the condition is more common in Caucasians.

Section 2

Signs and Symptoms of Crohn's Disease

Every patient may experience Crohn's disease a little bit differently.
We are available to assist you in navigating the most typical indications and symptoms of Crohn's disease. The specific GI tract impacted will determine the symptoms that you or a loved one may have.

Due to the chronic nature of Crohn's disease, patients may have flare-ups—periods when symptoms are particularly bad—followed by remissions—periods during which you may not have any symptoms at all.

Although it's critical to identify the symptoms of Crohn's disease, a diagnosis can only be verified by a medical professional. Please make an appointment with your doctor if you think you might have Inflammatory Bowel Diseases (IBD) so that a diagnosis and treatment plan can be developed.

GI Tract Inflammation

Any area of the gastrointestinal tract, from the mouth to the anus, can be impacted by Crohn's disease. Although each patient experiences symptoms differently, there are certain typical signs of GI tract inflammation brought on by Crohn's disease.

- Persistent diarrhea
- Rectal bleeding
- Urgent need to move bowels
- Abdominal cramps and pain
- Sensation of incomplete bowel evacuation
- Constipation, which can lead to bowel obstruction

Symptoms Beyond the Intestine

Inflammatory bowel disease (IBD) can cause systemic symptoms outside the GI tract that affect your overall health and your quality of life.

- Redness or pain in the eyes, or vision changes
- Mouth sores
- Swollen and painful joints

- Skin complications, such as bumps, sores, or rashes
- Fever
- Loss of appetite
- Weight Loss
- Fatigue
- Night sweats
- Loss of normal menstrual cycle
- Osteoporosis
- Kidney stones
- Rare liver complications, including primary sclerosing cholangitis and cirrhosis

Section 3

Causes of Crohn's Disease

An estimated one in every 100 Americans suffers from IBD. Sadly, little is known about the etiology of Crohn's disease at this time. For this reason, scientists studying Crohn's and colitis are trying to learn more about the condition and develop a treatment.

Crohn's Disease and the Immune System

In most cases, bacteria, viruses, fungus, and other foreign invaders are attacked and eliminated by the immune system of a human. When the immune system reacts normally, cells leave the circulation and enter the intestines, where they cause inflammation. Innocent bacteria in the gastrointestinal tract are normally shielded from immune system attacks.

In people with IBD:
- When these benign bacteria are misinterpreted by individuals with inflammatory bowel disease (IBD) as foreign invaders, the immune system reacts.
- The immunological response-induced inflammation does not go away. This results in intestinal wall thickening, ulceration, persistent inflammation, and ultimately Crohn's disease symptoms.

Genetic Factors

Since Crohn's disease tends to run in families, family members who have the condition or a close relative who has it are more likely to get it themselves. According to studies, 5% to 20% of individuals with IBD have a first-degree relative—a parent, child, or sibling—who also has the illness. Compared to ulcerative colitis, Crohn's disease carries a higher genetic risk.

Other Genetic Risk Factors
- When both parents have IBD, the likelihood of developing Crohn's disease

or ulcerative colitis is significantly increased.

- Those with eastern European ancestry, especially Jews of European heritage, are most likely to contract the illness.
- In African-American populations, the number of reported cases has grown recently.

Environmental Factors

Where you live appears to play a role in the development of Crohn's disease.

Here's where Crohn's disease is more common:

- Developed countries, rather than undeveloped countries
- Urban cities and towns, rather than rural areas
- Northern climates, rather than southern climates.

Section 4

Types of Crohn's Disease

It's critical to understand which area of your gastrointestinal tract is impacted if you receive a Crohn's disease diagnosis. Although Crohn's disease symptoms might differ from person to person, your specific kind of Crohn's affects the symptoms and potential consequences you may face.

Ileocolitis

The most prevalent type of Crohn's disease is this one. It affects the large intestine, also referred to as the colon, and the terminal ileum, which is the end of the small intestine. Possible symptoms include:

- Diarrhea and cramping
- Pain in the middle or lower right part of the abdomen
- Significant weight loss

Ileitis

This type of Crohn's affects only the ileum. Symptoms may include:

- Same as ileocolitis
- In severe cases, complications may include fistulas or inflammatory abscess in the right lower quadrant of the abdomen

Gastroduodenal Crohn's Disease

This type affects the stomach and the beginning of the small intestine, called the duodenum.

Symptoms may include:
- Nausea
- Vomiting
- Loss of appetite
- Weight loss

Jejunoileitis

This type is characterized by patchy areas of inflammation in the upper half of the small intestine, called the jejunum.

Symptoms may include:
- Mild to intense abdominal pain and cramps following meals
- Diarrhea

- Fistulas may form in severe cases or after prolonged periods of inflammation

Crohn's (Granulomatous) Colitis

This type affects only the colon, also known as the large intestine.

Symptoms may include:

- Diarrhea
- Rectal bleeding
- Disease around the anus, including abscess, fistulas and ulcers
- Skin lesions and joint pains are more common in this form of Crohn's than in others

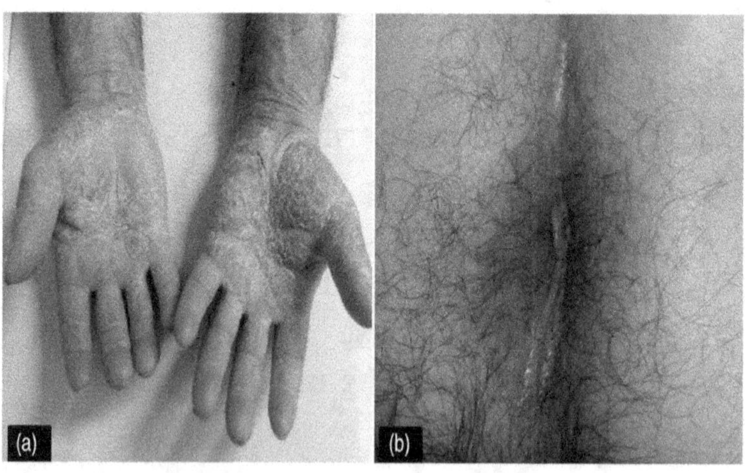

Section 5

Crohn's Disease Complications

While Crohn's disease is located in the GI tract, it can affect your overall health and cause more serious medical issues.

- Loss of appetite
- Weight loss
- Low energy and fatigue
- Delayed growth and development in children

In more severe cases, Crohn's disease can lead to serious complications.

- Fissures are tears in the lining of the anus, which can cause pain and bleeding especially during bowel movements.
- A fistula, caused by inflammation, is an abnormal channel that forms between one part of the intestine and another, or between the intestine and the bladder, vagina, or skin. Fistulas are most common in the anal area and require immediate medical attention.
- A stricture is a narrowing of the intestine as a result of chronic inflammation.

Section 6

Crohn's Disease Diagnosis and Testing

The symptoms of Crohn's disease might vary greatly from person to person. We will guide you through the diagnostic process step-by-step and provide you with updates.

The diagnosis of Crohn's disease cannot be made with a single test, and the symptoms of the illness are frequently confused with those of other illnesses, such as bacterial infections. Your medical professionals should assess your past medical history and utilize results from diagnostic tests to rule out any possible reasons for your symptoms. This procedure could take a while.

See your doctor right away if you think you or a loved one is exhibiting symptoms that could indicate Crohn's disease.

Initial Testing and Evaluation

A routine physical examination is the first step in diagnosing and treating your condition. In addition to talking with you, your doctor will inquire about your daily activities, family history, food and nutrition, and general health.

What to Expect

- To rule out other potential medical diseases and check for indicators of Crohn's disease, your doctor may prescribe diagnostic testing.
- Your blood and stool will probably be tested at a lab during your initial examinations.
- X-rays of the upper and lower GI tracts may be part of additional testing. A test that employs a contrast agent to provide a clearer, more detailed image of your gastrointestinal tract may be suggested by your physician. Every test has a different kind of contrast.
- Think about attending your appointments with a close friend or trusted family member. In addition to reducing your stress, this might assist

you recall details from your doctor in the future.

Communication Tips

- To ensure you don't overlook anything crucial, make a note of your symptoms and bring it to your appointments.
- Consult your medical team about the appropriate test for you, and get information on cost sharing from your insurance company.

Endoscopy and Imaging

In order to examine your intestine and GI tract, your doctor might advise further testing. Even though these tests are more intrusive and could seem scary, your healthcare providers will take care to minimize any discomfort because they are frequently performed in an outpatient setting.

Endoscopy

A tiny camera attached to the end of a lit tube allows your doctor to take a close look inside your colon during an endoscopy.

The following endoscopies are used to screen for Crohn's disease:

- During a colonoscopy, a flexible, lighted tube is inserted through your anus opening to allow medical professionals to inspect the colon, which is the lowest portion of your large intestine.
- Using a flexible, illuminated tube that is passed through your mouth, down your esophagus, into your stomach, and all the way down to the duodenum—the first part of your small intestine—an upper endoscopy allows medical professionals to view the gastrointestinal system from the top down.

Bowel preparation is required for colonoscopies. Discuss preparation strategies and easy preparation hacks with your healthcare team.

Biopsy

During a colonoscopy or endoscopy, your doctor might wish to take a biopsy from your colon or another part of your digestive system. A tiny sample of tissue from the inside of the gut is taken out during the biopsy in order to be tested and examined further.

- In a pathology lab, your biopsied tissue will be examined and examined for any diseases. Screening for colorectal cancer also involves biopsies.
- Although a biopsy may seem frightening, thanks to advancements in medicine, the process is now almost painless.

Chromoendoscopy

In order to search for polyps or precancerous alterations during a colonoscopy, your doctor might wish to employ this approach.

- A blue liquid dye is injected into the colon during a chromoendoscopy in order to identify and emphasize minute alterations in the intestinal lining.
- After that, polyps can be removed or biopsied.
- Blue bowel motions are a common side effect of this therapy.

Small Intestine Imaging

These tests are intended to look at areas of your gut that a colonoscopy or endoscopy cannot easily view. They function by using a drinkable oral contrast that is visible on a computed tomography (CT), magnetic resonance imaging (MRI), or fluoroscopic X-ray.

- These examinations may also be referred to as enteroclysis or enterography.
- A tiny, pill-sized camera that takes images of your small intestine and colon as it passes through your GI tract might be given to you to swallow by your doctor. Later on, the camera comes out during a bowel movement.
- To observe parts of the intestine that are difficult to access, a balloon endoscopy could be required.

Communication Tips

- Find out from your medical professionals what to anticipate from the procedure and whether there are any potential hazards.
- The majority of Crohn's disease testing takes place in an outpatient

environment. If you want some company and peace of mind while driving, think about having a friend or relative do the driving.

Section 7

Crohn's Disease Treatment Options

You may maintain control over your illness and enjoy a fulfilling life by utilizing a variety of therapy modalities. Recall that no single treatment is universally effective for every patient. Every patient has a unique scenario, and each one requires a different course of treatment.

Crohn's disease and other types of inflammatory bowel disease (IBD) can be treated with medication, clinical trials, dietary and nutritional changes, and occasionally surgery to remove or repair damaged GI tract sections.

Medication

The goal of Crohn's disease medication is to reduce the aberrant inflammatory response that your immune system is producing, which is the source of your symptoms. In addition to providing relief from common symptoms like fever, diarrhea, and pain, suppressing inflammation promotes the healing of your intestinal tissues.

Medication can be used to reduce the frequency of symptom flare-ups in addition to managing and suppressing symptoms (inducing remission) (maintaining remission). Periods of remission can be prolonged and times when symptoms flare up can be decreased with appropriate medication administered gradually. Nowadays, there are several different kinds of medications used to treat Crohn's disease.

Combination Therapy

A healthcare professional may in some cases advise adding a complementary therapy to the original therapy in order to maximize its efficacy. Combination therapy, for instance, can involve adding a biologic in addition to an immunomodulator. Combination therapy has advantages and disadvantages, just like any other type of therapy. Combining treatments can improve how well IBD is treated, but there may be a higher chance of toxicity and other side effects. The best course of action for your particular set of medical needs will be determined by your healthcare practitioner.

Clinical Trials

A lot of people don't know that they can treat their IBD by enrolling in a research study. Researchers discover novel approaches to enhance treatments and quality of life through clinical trials. Only through clinical trials can new and better treatment choices for patients become available. Clinical trials are one of the last phases of a drawn-out and meticulous research process. To identify a trial that might be a good fit for you and to learn more about clinical trials, visit the Clinical Trials Community.

Diet & Nutrition

Even though adverse food reactions may not be the cause of Crohn's disease, paying close attention to your diet can help minimize symptoms, replenish depleted nutrients, and encourage healing.

Maintaining a healthy diet is crucial for those with Crohn's disease because the condition frequently causes appetite reduction in addition to an increase in the body's requirement for energy. Furthermore, common Crohn's symptoms like diarrhea might hinder your body's absorption of water, vitamins, minerals, protein, fat, and carbohydrates.

Soft, bland foods are often less uncomfortable for many people who have Crohn's disease flare-ups than spicy or high-fiber foods. If you are diagnosed as lactose intolerant, your diet can still be flexible and should consist of a range of foods from all food categories, but your doctor will probably advise you to limit your dairy intake.

Surgery

Up to two-thirds to three-quarters of individuals with Crohn's disease will need surgery at some time in their lives, even with appropriate medicine and diet. Surgery can restore your highest quality of life and save a piece of your GI tract, even though it cannot cure Crohn's disease.

When medication is no longer able to control your symptoms, or if you develop an intestinal blockage, fistula, or fissure, surgery becomes necessary. Anastomosis, or the joining of the two ends of healthy bowel, follows the removal of the diseased segment of the colon (resection) in most cases. Even while these treatments could make your symptoms go away for a long time, Crohn's disease usually returns in later life.

Key things to know about Surgery:
- Studies have revealed that 18% of Crohn's patients may eventually need surgery over a 5-year period. In recent years, there has been a notable decrease in this percentage.
- Depending on the cause, severity, and location of the condition, several operations may be carried out.
- About 31% of Crohn's disease patients might need a second resection ten years after their initial one.

Section 8

Making Knowledgeable Choices (Consult Your Physician)

You're not the only one who finds it difficult to understand the plethora of available drugs and treatments! Because IBD is so complicated, it's critical to discuss the advantages and disadvantages of every treatment option with your physician.

Questions to Ask Your Doctor

Upon receiving a Crohn's disease diagnosis, it's normal to experience uncertainty and anxiety. Numerous parts of your life may be impacted by Crohn's disease, and these effects may vary over time.

Studying as much as you can about Crohn's disease is the greatest approach to get ready for life with the condition. You can initiate conversation with your healthcare professional by asking these questions. Your ability to manage your condition and live the life you desire will improve with increased knowledge about Crohn's disease.

Knowing Crohn's disease, inquire with your physician about the following:
- Why do people get Crohn's?
- What are Crohn's disease symptoms and indicators?
- Which kind of Crohn's disease am Ihaving?
- How can I keep an eye on my health?
- How can I tell if I'm experiencing a flare-up?
- When my Crohn's disease is in remission, how will I know?

Ask your doctor the following questions regarding relationships and lifestyle:
- How is Crohn's going to impact my travel, employment, and fitness?
- Must I change the way I eat? If yes, how?
- What impact will Crohn's illness have on pregnancy and family planning?
- How will my disease affect other people?

Ask your doctor the following questions regarding the types of exploring treatments:

- How is the treatment for Crohn's disease administered?
- What are the benefits and drawbacks of the treatment?
- What types of adverse effects am I likely to experience from my medication?
- Will I need to have surgery? If so, what is involved in that?
- What more therapies are offered?

Ask your doctor the following questions regarding managing the disease:

- What can I do to stop flare-ups?
- When ought I to visit the doctor?
- How may I reduce my symptoms at home?

Stress-Relieving Advice

- Bring writing supplies to your appointment so you may jot down terms and any issues you want to discuss with your physician.
- Inquire with your physician or nurse about the most effective way to follow up with them between visits.